Practice Guidelines

For Diagnostic, Treatment, and Related Support Services for Persons with Developmental Disabilities and Serious Behavioral Problems

William I. Gardner, Ph.D. (Panel Chairperson)
Anton Dosen, M. D., Ph.D.
Dorothy M. Griffiths, Ph.D.
Robert King, M. D.

With Technical Support by
Andre Lapointe, Ph.D.

NADD An association for persons with developmental disabilities and mental health needs.

132 Fair Street
Kingston, NY 12401

LCCN: 2006936144
ISBN: 1-57256-046-0

Printed in the United States Of America

Contents

Preface 1

PART A: INTRODUCTION

Section 1.
Need for and Process of Development of Practice Guidelines 3

Section 2.
Definition of Serious Behavior Problems .6

Section 3.
Serious Behavior Problems and Psychiatric Disorders:
Differential Diagnosis and Treatment Implications 8

Section 4.
Serious Behavior Problems and Physical Illness:
Differential Diagnosis and Treatment Implications 10

Section 5.
Serious Behavior Problems and Genetic Syndromes and Conditions:
Differential Diagnosis and Treatment Implications 12

Section 6.
Serious Behavior Problems at Different Developmental Levels 14

Section 7.
Focus of Assessment and Related Treatment Process 16

PART B: PRACTICE GUIDELINES

Guideline 1.Comprehensive Biopsychosocial Assessments 26
1a.Purpose and Content of Assessments 26
1b.Integration of Assessment Results 29
1c.Composition and Credentials of Assessment Staff. 29
1d.Settings in Which Assessment and Related Activities Occur . . . 30

Guideline 2.Integrated Treatment and Support Plan 32
2a.Hypothesis-based Interventions 32
2b.Content of CITSP 32
2c.Components of CITSP 33
2d.Empirically-based Interventions 34

Guideline 3.Behavioral Crisis Deceleration Strategies and Crisis Management Supports 34
3a.Content of DSCM 35
3b.Review and Modification of DSCM 35
3c. Continuum of Crisis Services in Natural Environments 36

Guideline 4.Assessment of CITSP Effectiveness 37
4a. Objective Data Systems 37
4b.Functions of Data Systems 37
4c.Ongoing Nature of Assessment 37

Guideline 5.Comprehensive Individualized Treatment and Related Support Plan Services 37
5a. Types of CITSP Services. 37
5b.Contexts of Treatment and Related Support Services 38
5c. Targets of CITSP Support Services 38
5d.Delivery of CITSP Services. 38

Guideline 6.Coordination of Treatment and Related Support Services . . . 39
6a. Treatment Plan Coordinator 39
6b. Functions of Treatment Plan Coordinator. 39
6c. Caseload of Treatment Plan Coordinator 40
6d. Duration of Services of Treatment Plan Coordinator 41

Guideline 7. Approaches to Delivery of Core and Related Services 41
7a. Service Agency or Consortium of Service Agencies 41
7b. Seamless Service Delivery 41
7c. Specific Responsibilities for Coordination of Services 41
7d. Services and Roles 42
Summary. 42

References 44

Preface

These Practice Guidelines were prepared by a panel of professionals with extensive training, research, and clinical experiences in serving persons with developmental disabilities who present with serious behavior problems (SBPs). Funding and technical support were provided by the PREM-TGC (The Programme Regional D'Expertise Multidisciplinare en Troubles Graves du Comportements) of Quebec, Canada. The Panel consisted of:

- William I. Gardner, Ph.D., Emeritus Professor, University of Wisconsin-Madison, USA, Former Vice President and Board of Directors, National Association for the Dually Diagnosed (Panel Chairperson),
- Anton Dosen, M.D., Ph.D., Professor, Nijegen University, The Netherlands, Past President and current Board, European Association of Mental Health and Mental Retardation
- Dorothy Griffiths, Ph.D., Professor, Brock University, Ontario, Canada, Past President and Board of Directors, National Association for the Dually Diagnoses
- Robert King, M.D., Psychiatrist, North Bay Psychiatric Hospital, Ontario, Canada

Andre Lapointe, Ph.D., Psychology, PREM-TGC, provided invaluable technical support to the Panel and served as staff liaison between the PREM agency and the Panel.

In developing these Practice Guidelines, the Panel recognized that limited resources or current administrative and service agency structures present in various local, regional or national settings might impede attainment of all components of these Guidelines. Nonetheless, the objectives that guided the Panel were *those of identifying needs of persons with SBPs and of describing the types of services, personnel, and agency structures required to address these needs.* As such, these Practice Guidelines offer (a) a template for use by governmental and private agencies at local, regional, provincial, and national levels to evaluate the status of current clinical and related support services and (b) a blueprint for modifying or expanding existing services to insure that unmet needs are addressed.

The reader should distinguish the Practice Guidelines described in this paper from specific *treatment* guidelines that typically are defined as those that "provide specific recommendations about treatments to be offered to clients" (Reed, McLaughlin, & Newman, 2002, p. 1042). The National Guidelines Clearinghouse provides a listing of over 100 such guidelines in the behavioral health area (www.guideline.gov). Rush and Frances (2000) provide an example of treatment guidelines for psychiatric and behavioral problems presented by persons with mental retardation.

Part A: Introduction

SECTION 1. Need for and Process of Development of Practice Guidelines

The chronic nature of SBPs restricts the person's inclusion in a range of developmentally appropriate and desirable social, educational, vocational, and recreational experiences. Such restrictions are inconsistent with normalization goals of social inclusion, open access to natural community options, and free expression of personal choices and preferences. The presence of these SBPs also may pose a significant burden on the family and other caregivers who support the person in residential and day services (Jacobson, Holburn, & Mulick, 2002).

In consideration of the wide array of possible biomedical and psychosocial conditions that may contribute to the development and chronic recurrence of SBPs in persons with intellectual and other developmental disabilities (DD), a comprehensive and coordinated array of core diagnostic, treatment, and related supports is required for optimal remediation and management of these problems.

Although diagnostic, treatment, case management, and related support services may be available in generic mental health, developmental disabilities, health, education and social service agencies, these services are commonly informed by treatment models lacking the comprehensiveness of a developmentally sensitive biopsychosocial understanding of SBPs. Furthermore, these services typically are challenged by a shortage of specially trained and experienced staff and related specialized services dedicated to providing supports specifically for individuals with DD. The extensive clinical experiences of Panel Members suggest that a clinical service focus on a narrow and limited range of biomedical, psychological, or social environmental conditions frequently results in the excessive and inappropriate use of psychotropic medication and restrictive behavioral procedures provided in attempts to manage the SBPs. Finally, these generic services typically lack the capacity to offer the comprehensive and coordinated life span supports that are required to insure that the SBPs are optimally treated at the time of initial occurrence or recurrence to insure that the person's quality of life experiences are enhanced and maintained. As a result, significant biomedical, psychological, and social conditions that contribute to the occurrence, severity, and the chronic nature of a person's SBPs may be unrecognized and untreated (Griffiths & Gardner, 2002a, 2002b; Jacobson, Holburn, & Mulick, 2002; Jacobson, Mulick, & Holburn, 2002).

These *Practice Guidelines* address the essential characteristics of these core services and supports and are based on the premise that all citizens including those with developmental disabilities should indeed have those services and supports needed to expertly diagnose and treat the conditions that produce and maintain each person's SBPs. Further, these services and supports should be individually-centered, available in or to the community in which the person resides, and offered in a manner that meets the personal needs and desires of each individual in the most normalizing manner possible. Successful attainment of these service objectives is best realized when there is a collaborative fusion of developmental disabilities and mental health expertise with community and regional generic health, educational, and social services. Thus, all core services and related supports are designed to support the personal goals and preferences of each person served (Griffiths & Gardner, 2002a,b.)

Several early revisions of these Practice Guidelines were based on feedback from a range of professionals who provided supports for persons with SBPs in the province of Quebec, Canada. Additionally, more recent revisions resulted from audience feedback obtained following presentations of the Guidelines during meetings of the European Association on Mental Health In Mental Retardation held in Barcelona, Spain on October 8, 2005 and the NADD International Congress held in Boston on March 16, 2006.

In the sections to follow, definition of SBPs in persons with developmental disabilities precedes brief discussion of a number of potential comorbid conditions that, when present, may serve significant roles in occurrence and severity of a person's SBPs. Knowledge of the possible influences of these on a person's SBPs offers a valuable basis for:

(a) Selection of the types and essential features of specialized diagnostic, treatment, and related support services needed to most successfully address the potentially multiple biomedical and psychosocial conditions that control a person's SBPs,

(b) Description of essential features of objective data observation, recording, and evaluation systems to track treatment program progress and outcome effectiveness,

(c) Identification of the professional qualifications and functions of persons needed to deliver these services, and

(d) Selection of service delivery models that best insure access to these.

These *Practice Guidelines* represent current thinking as determined through an analysis of pertinent conceptual and empirical literatures and the integration of knowledge gained with clinical practice expertise and person-centered values (Dosen, 2005 a, b; Gardner & Hunter, 2003; Griffiths, Stavrakaki, & Summers, 2002; Jacobson, Holburn, & Mulick, 2002; Jacobson, Mulick, & Holburn, 2002). As these Guidelines are aspirational in intent rather than being viewed as final standards of service practice, the authors anticipate that these will be refined over time as North American and international audiences offer additional feedback.

SECTION 2. Definition of Serious Behavior Problems

Behavioral acts such as physical aggression, property destruction, self-injury, pica, and related agitated/disruptive episodes are defined as serious by a person's social environments due to the (a) *frequency* of occurrence, (b) *severity* (the potential for physical or psychological harm to the person or others or to property), and (c) *durability* over time and situations of the behaviors. Some problem behaviors may be of low frequency but of high intensity and thus viewed as serious in nature. Others behaviors may be viewed as serious, even if of relatively low intensity, due to the high and persistent frequency of occurrence (Emerson, 2001). In considering harm to the person, others, or property, attention is given to a number of areas including degree of destruction of materials, degree of interference with social interactions, frequency and degree of interference with learning and rehabilitation, degree of exposure to aversive or restrictive procedures, limitation of access to community services, reduction of the person's civic rights (e.g., being place in jail), and potential for restriction of a person's freedom through hospitalization or institutionalization (O'Brien, 2003).

Persons with SBPs represent a heterogeneous group both in age and in types and levels of disabilities. In fact, as SBPs typically develop gradually over a period of months and years and occur in an increasing number of life situations, it is not unusual for behavioral problems to appear during the early developmental years and to increase in frequency and severity during a person's ensuing adolescent and young adult years (Emerson, 2001; Richardson, Koller, & Katz, 1985). As a result, significantly different individual needs are present that require highly individualized clinical attention.

There is general agreement among writers that problem behaviors cannot be reduced to a single psychiatric or other medical diagnostic category (Pary 2005). Although SBPs may in fact develop in the absence of coexisting psychiatric, other medical, genetic and related disorders, the potential influence of biomedical conditions when present either may be overlooked or, in some instances, be inappropriately viewed as the major cause with inadequate attention given to other influences of a psychosocial nature. The following brief discussion explores these possible biomedical influences and the resulting need for a comprehensive case formation approach that gives adequate attention both to these and the possible interactions with psychosocial conditions that may influence development and occurrence of SBPs.

SECTION 3. Serious Behavior Problems and Psychiatric Disorders: Differential Diagnosis and Treatment Implications

A number of writers have noted that SBPs occur with increased frequency in persons who also present with symptoms of one or more psychiatric disorders. (Moss, Emerson, Kierman, Turner, Hatton, & Alborz, 2000; Reiss & Aman, 1998). Table 1 includes a few examples of psychiatric symptoms reported to demonstrate this relationship. Changes in frequency and severity of SBPs in the absence of apparent changes in environmental, psychological, or physical illness conditions may suggest the presence of these and other similar influential psychiatric symptoms such as heightened levels of irritability, hallucinations, or a dysphoric mood. In instances of a possible relationship of these to SBPs, informed clinical practice would dictate that the psychiatric influence be identified and treatment directed to these psychiatric conditions. Successful treatment of the implicated psychiatric illness and related symptoms would in turn result in reduction or elimination of those SBPs influenced by these conditions.

It is highly unusual, however, that psychiatric disorders represent the sole causes of a person's SBPs. Most typically, various symptoms of psychiatric disorders combine with environmental and psychological conditions to contribute to the frequency of occurrence, severity levels, and variability in frequency and severity of SBPs. As later described in Part B, symptoms of a psychiatric illness may serve multiple roles in influencing these SBPs. Clinical reports suggest that the magnitude of influence of co-occurring psychiatric disorders on frequency and severity levels and on likelihood of recurrence of a person's SBPs may range from minor to major.

Psychiatric Features	References
Flashbacks	Ryan (1994; 2000)
Emotional overarousal	Sovner et al. (1993); Tsiouris (2001); Vitiello, Spreat, & Behar (1989); Vitiello & Stoff (1997)
Delusional cognitions	Cole & Gardner (1990)
Delirious state	Gedye (1997)
Anxiety symptoms	Moss et al. (2000)

Table 1. Studies illustrating influence of psychiatric symptoms on SBPs.

Even more complex problems may emerge when SBPs influence occurrence of a psychiatric disorder. This may result when a person's SBPs create severe conflict with the social surroundings, thus leading to social isolation, maltreatment, recurring restraints, or excessive and inappropriate use of medication. These chronic stress conditions may disrupt biological and psychological regulation systems and assume an influential role in precipitating a mental illness.

In summary, while co-occurring psychiatric disorders may *contribute* to the onset, severity, and variability in frequency and severity over time and settings of a person's SBPs, psychiatric conditions most typically exert their influence in combination with concurrent physical illness and psychological conditions of the person as these effects in turn interact with features of the person's physical and social environments. A diagnostic and treatment case formulation approach thus is required to insure identification of (a) the specific roles assumed by psychiatric conditions in influencing SBPs, (b) the magnitude of effects of these psychiatric conditions on SBPs when combined with other physical illness, psychological, and environmental influences, and (c) the potential role that SBPs may assume in contributing to occurrence of a psychiatric illness.

SECTION 4. Serious Behavior Problems and Physical Illness: Differential Diagnosis and Treatment Implications

A range of acute and chronic physical illnesses or pathologies may create distressful psychophysiological experiences such as pain, discomfort, fatigue, anxiety, excitability, irritability, and related mood deviations. These medical conditions include such illnesses as chronic headaches, menstrual discomfort, middle ear infections, allergic reactions, skin disorders, cardiac difficulties, sleep irregularities, constipation, gastrointestinal distress, seizure disorders, and tooth infections as well as the side effects of psychotropic and other medications. Additionally, dysfunctions of specific central nervous system areas as illustrated by lesions of the prefrontal cortex and epilepsy (particularly in persons with uncontrolled seizures) may represent significant risk factors for occurrence of impulsive episodes of SBPs. In fact, changes in frequency of occurrence and in severity levels of SBPs in the absence of changes in apparent psychiatric, environmental, or psychological causes may suggest the presence of co-occurring physical illnesses or pathologies.

A number of studies have supported the thesis that an increase in a person's distress level created by these conditions may influence occurrence, severity levels, and variability in occurrence and severity of SBPs (See Table 2 for references that offer illustrations of these influences). As described later in Part B, these personal experiences may serve multiple roles in influencing occurrence, severity, and persistence of SBPs.

In these instances, informed clinical practice dictates that the physical illness condition be identified and appropriate treatment directed to the physical illness or pathology itself. Successful treatment or management of these medical conditions may remove or reduce the pathology and the related personal distress levels and thus influence reduction in frequency or severity levels of related SBPs. It is quite unusual, however, that chronically occurring SBPs would completely disappear following successful management or treatment of the implicated physical illness or condition if other contributing environmental, psychological, or psychiatric influences remain unidentified and unaddressed.

It should be noted that some medical conditions present on a cyclic basis and may be of relatively short duration for any given occurrence, e.g., premenstrual distress or allergies. As these conditions may be masked by the person's SBPs, the comprehensive assessment will require careful analysis of variations in frequency and severity of SBPs that are not accounted for by other conditions.

In summary, while co-occurring physical illnesses or disorders may contribute to the occurrence, severity, and variability in frequency and severity of SBPs, these conditions typically exert their influence in interaction with possible co-occurring psychiatric, psychological, and environmental features. A diagnostic and treatment case formulation approach that recognizes the interactive effects of a physical illness is required to insure interface of all contributors in formulating an appropriate individualized treatment and support plan for a person's SBPs.

Physical Illness Conditions	**References**
Acute and chronic medical conditions such as itchy eyes, constipation, earache, boils, eczema	Peine et al. (1995)
Iron deficiency anemia	Tu, Shafey, & VanDewetering (1994)
Sleep irregularities	Brylweski & Wiggs (1999); O"Reilly (1995)
Seizure medication side effects such as irritability	Kalachnik, Hanzel, Harder, Bauernfeind, & Engstrom (1995)
Frontal and temporal lobe seizures	Creaby, Warner, Jamil, & Jawad (1993); Tucker, Price, Johnson, & McAllister (1986)
Pain secondary to dental abscess or menstruation	Gardner & Whalen (1996)
Psychotropic medication side effects such as fatigue, anxiety, irritability, mania, and excitability	Gardner & Sovner (1994); Friedman, Kastner, Plummer, Ruiz, & Henning (1992)

Table 2. Studies illustrating influence of physical illness and pathologies on SBPs.

SECTION 5. Serious Behavior Problems and Genetic Syndromes and Conditions: Differential Diagnosis and Treatment Implications

A number of writers, as illustrated in Table 3, have noted that various behavioral and emotional features occur with greater frequency among persons with specific genetic disorders relative to comparison groups without these disorders. The term "behavioral phenotypes" is used to describe this relationship and refers to "the heightened probability or likelihood that people with a given syndrome will exhibit certain behavioral and developmental sequelae relative to those without the syndrome" (Dykens, 1996, p. 523). Persons with such syndromes as Cornelia de Lange, Cri-Du-Chat, Fragile X, Praeder-Willi, Retts, Smith-Magenis, Tourette's, and Williams present a range of neuropsychological features that serve as significant risk conditions for occurrence and severity of SBPs. These conditions include pervasive hyperactivity, ritualistic behaviors, impulsivity, fatigue and related irritability associated with sleep disorders, anxiety, attention deficits, overarousal in response to minor environmental stimuli, and emotional lability with cycles of positive and negative affect (Anderson & Ernst, 1994; Dykens, 1996; Dykens, Hodapp, & Finucane, 2000; Griffiths & King, 2004; Griffiths & Watson, 2004; Tuinier & Verhoeven, 1993). To illustrate, persons with syndromes such as Lesch-Nyhan, Smith-Magenis, Prader-Willi, and Cornelia de Lange are at increased risk for SBPs involving aggressive and self-injurious acts.

Genetic Syndromes	References
Lesch-Nyhan syndrome	Anderson & Ernst (1994)
Fragile-X syndrome	Barnhill (2001)
Gilles de la Tourette syndrome	Comings & Comings (1985); King (1999); Robertson, Trimble, & Lees (1989)
Williams syndrome	Einfeld, Tonge, & Forio (1997)

Table 3. Studies illustrating influence of features of persons with various genetic syndromes on SBPs.

In summary, co-occurring genetic syndromes may result in a number of neurological and related psychological features that may serve various roles in increasing the risk of occurrence of SBPs. As these features vary both in the magnitude of effects on occurrence and severity level of SBPs and in the manner in which these interact with other physical illness, psychiatric, psychological, and environmental conditions, a diagnostic and treatment case formulation approach that recognizes the potential interactive effects of conditions associated with genetic syndromes is required to insure interface of all contributors in formulating an appropriate individualized treatment and support plan for a person's SBPs.

SECTION 6. Serious Behavior Problems at Different Developmental Levels

Persons at different levels of psychosocial development may process or interpret situations differently and thus may respond with different behaviors. The child development literature indicates that at each developmental level the typically developing child acquires particular adaptive behaviors under favorable conditions as well as maladaptive behaviors under unfavorable circumstances. Briefly, an infant may react to a stressful situation with excessive irritability, head banging, temper tantrums, and destructiveness. A toddler may react to stressful conditions in an oppositional and defiant manner or with hyperactivity and acts of impulsive aggression. During school age, a child may demonstrate compulsive and obsessive behaviors or may exhibit aggressive or destructive behaviors. During the assessment of persons with developmental disabilities who present with SBPs, it may be observed that individuals at particular levels of cognitive and related language impairments may demonstrate maladaptive behaviors similar to those observed in the typically developing child at various stages of the normal developmental process. In summary, this developmental progression suggests that the manner in which the child with intellectual disabilities processes unfavorable or stressful circumstances and the coping reactions that follow differ at different developmental levels similar to that observed in typically developing children at comparable developmental levels.

At each developmental level, a person's psychosocial needs are different and must be met for typical progression to a later stage. If demands are encountered that are beyond the person's developmental capabilities, maladaptive behavior is likely to occur. To illustrate, a young child, or a person at a profound level of psychological developmental impairment who also has severe problems of regulation of basic physiological needs, such as sleep-awake rhythm, eating, digestion, and with difficulties of processing sensory stimuli, will demonstrate considerable difficulties of processing and coping with any unfavorable circumstances such as intense sensory stimuli and change of evironment. Maladaptive behavioral reactions are likely to occur. If a person has difficulty with forming and maintaining attachments, it would be expected that the person would have difficulty coping with environmental demands due to the person's excessive security needs with the result that maladaptive behaviors will occur in response to the demands. In a similar manner, an individual with difficulties in development of personal autonomy would view situations that require more independence as threatening and likely would cope with these with such maladaptive behaviors as excessive attention seeking.

For a better understanding of behavioral features at particular developmental levels, the concept of personality development has been offered. Personality has been conceptualized as a result of cognitive, social, and emotional development (Greenspan, 1997; Harris, 1998). The developmental levels attained within the cognitive, social, and emotional domains define personality developmental level. Personality developmental level reflects the basic psychosocial needs that require satisfaction in order to develop the motivation for development and use of adaptive behaviors by means of which the person interacts with the social and physical environments. As a result of positive feedback from the surroundings, harmonious and healthy development is stimulated. In instances in which environmental circumstances do not meet basic personal needs, inappropriate motivational conditions occur that influence maladaptive behaviors. In situations that involve durable or recurrent stressful events, the inappropriate behaviors may become the major or sole interactions with the environment.

In summary, a person's developmental levels (cognitive, social, emotional, and personality traits) represent critical features that influence the manner in which the person processes and interprets unfavorable circumstances as well as the resulting behavioral reactions exhibited. See Dosen (2004), Dosen (2005a, b) and Forehand and Wierson (1993) for elaboration of these developmental processes.

SECTION 7. Focus of the Assessment and Related Treatment Process

Recurring acts of SBPs are best understood when viewed within a dynamic interactive context consisting of (a) *instigating conditions*, (b) *central processing conditions*, and (c) *maintaining* conditions. The specific influences of the antecedent *instigating* conditions on the behavioral acts are determined by the transactions between these and a person's psychobiological and psychological *central processing* features. As noted above, these central processing features include and reflect a person's developmental levels of functioning (cognitive, social, emotional, personality). The effects produced by a behavioral occurrence on a person's current motivational condition(s) that provided the impetus for the behavior, in turn, determine the likelihood of recurrence of the SPBs. These effects represent the reinforcing or maintaining conditions that contribute to the habit strength (likelihood of recurrence when again exposed to similar antecedent conditions) of the SBP. This sequence of events is as follows: Instigating events ⇔ Central Processing influences ⇒ Behavioral act ⇔ Environmental and Personal Consequences.

As noted in the following sections, selection of specific treatment and management approaches for a person's SBPs is based on diagnostic information about conditions in each of these three influential contexts and the manner in which these interact. *These instigating, central processing, and maintaining conditions that determine the occurrence, severity level, variability, and pervasiveness of a person's SBPs thus become the targets of treatments.* As assessment results may implicate multiple and individually unique sources of biomedical and psychosocial influences on a person's SBPs, a number of different interventions may be required to address these multiple sets of controlling influences.

A brief description of each context is provided.

CONTEXT 1: Instigating Conditions

Serious behavioral acts or episodes do not occur randomly or haphazardly. Rather, SBPs occur selectively under specific and individually salient antecedent conditions that create or intensify experiences of personal distress. These distress-producing antecedents consist of influential instigating conditions that may arise from a person's *social and physical environmental settings* in which these SBPs occur (e.g., instructional demands, conflict with peers, blocking of ritualistic or compulsive routines, invasion of personal space). These environmental antecedents may combine with current *psychological and biomedical stimulus* features of the person that may change the influence of these environmental conditions (e.g., high arousal level, anger, pain-related distress, deprivation state, dysphoric mood). These instigating stimulus conditions are highly specific to each person (McComas, Hoch, Paone, & El-Roy, 2000) and when present represent risk factors for SBPs for that person. In some instances the instigating conditions may arise from internal states as illustrated in some episodes of self-injury that occur independent of environmental instigation.

The following provide illustrations of the additive instigating effects of different sources of antecedent conditions:

> A child may engage in episodes of severe self-injury in response to an instructional directive provided by a teacher (environmental social instigating condition). It also may be observed that on some occasions following teacher directives these self-injurious episodes (SIBs) become more severe in intensity and episode duration. Additional analysis may reveal that these more severe and lengthy episodes occur when the child also is experiencing heightened levels of irritability presumed to result from medication prescribed for a seizure disorder (internal psychological instigating conditions resulting from aberrant medical conditions). The increase in severity level and duration of SIB episodes may be the initial diagnostic cue that some instigating influences in addition to the teacher's instructional directive are present. These combined instigating influences require identification to insure development of an intervention plan that addresses both sources of antecedent influence.

As a second illustration:

> The aggressive acts of a young man with a bipolar disorder in response to unwanted directives from parents (social environmental instigating conditions) may be observed to increase in *frequency* of occurrence (e.g., from one time per day to five times per day) and *severity* (e.g., from minor intensity with minimal likelihood of physical harm to major intensity with high likelihood of physical harm to self) during episodes of mania, hypomania, or depression (internally-based instigating conditions resulting from distress-producing psychiatric conditions). These diagnostic insights relating to multiple and interactive sources of instigating influences provide the basis for selection of treatments that address both the psychiatric condition and the person's mode of responding to parental directives.

CONTEXT 2: Central Processing Features

The level of risk and the particular pattern of behaviors that may occur when exposed to individually salient conditions of instigation are related to the type, number, and strength of a person's uniquely individual *psychobiological and psychological* central-processing features that serve as mediating influences. The specific components of these psychobiological and psychological systems reflect the *current developmental* features of a person within different dimensions of functioning (cognitive, social, emotional, personality). To emphasize, these features determine both the manner in which the instigating conditions will be processed by the person and the nature of the resulting coping behavioral reactions. An understanding of a person's current mediating central processing features will assist the clinician in answering the question of why one person would be at increased risk for occurrence of SBPs when another person would be at minimal or no risk when both are exposed to such similar antecedent conditions as peer provocation, staff instructional directives, or heightened levels of anger arousal.

PSYCHOBIOLOGICAL FEATURES. Aspects of the *psychobiological* central processing system that represent risk factors for SBPs consist of features produced by or associated with (a) neurological and related neurochemical abnormalities (b) psychiatric disorders and symptoms (c) other medical abnormalities and (d) conditions associated with various genetic syndromes (Barnhill, 1999; Tuinier & Verhoeven, 1993; Gedye, 1997; Dykens et al., 2000). To illustrate, a person's neurological and biochemical abnormalities may result in an inclination for generalized affective overarousal (hyperexcitability, hyperirritability), even to seemingly minor conditions of threat or provocation. As a second illustration, related impairments in the processes of modulating states of overarousal may result in the person remaining in an overaroused state for extended periods and being at increased risk for engaging in exaggerated impulsive problem behaviors when exposed to such seemingly minor sources of provocation as a directive from a caregiver (Bradley, 2000). These abnormalities are seen with increased frequency and severity among persons with more severe intellectual disabilities. Additionally, similar personal features are reported in persons with intellectual disabilities who also present with various psychiatric and personality disorders, acute and chronic physical illnesses, and various genetic syndromes.

Persons with psychiatric disorders also present with other more discrete features that may serve as mediating risk influences on SBPs. Various *mood/affective* (e.g., irritability, dysphoria, anxiety, emotional lability), *cognitive* (e.g. delusional thought content), *perceptual* (e.g., auditory and visual hallucinations), and related symptoms associated with major mental disorders and various personality disorders and traits may influence the personal meaning or function of incoming instigating stimulus events. To illustrate, a person may have a tendency to view the actions of others in a suspicious or threatening manner. These and similar paranoid traits are reported to occur with some frequency in persons with intellectual disabilities who engage in SBPs (Bouras & Drummond, 1992; Reiss, 1992). This cognitive and related emotional view of the actions of others will influence the information-processing activities involved in the encoding and interpretation of social events and, in turn, will influence the selection and evaluation of alternatives to SBPs as possible means of coping with the perceived sources of threat. As a result, these processing difficulties in combination with the person's acquired habits of SBPs are likely to result in an SBP episode directed at (e.g., aggression) or in response to (e.g., self-injurious behaviors) the perceived source of threat. This scenario emphasizes the dynamic interactions between instigating events and a person's unique central processing features.

PSYCHOLOGICAL DEVELOPMENTAL FEATURES. The second category of central processing risk conditions for occurrence of SBPs consists of two groups of *psychological* features. These features reflect the person's current *developmental levels* in each of the cognitive, social, emotional, and broader personality areas of functioning. The initial grouping consists of psychological developmental features of a cognitive, emotional, motivational, and behavioral nature that, due to their *presence or excessive* nature, increase the risk for occurrence of SBPs. This grouping of risk influences is illustrated by features such as the following, that reflect differing developmental learning influences: (a) presence of strong inclination to engage in SBPs, (b) a cognitive hostile attributional bias, (c) other cognitive distortions (for example, a belief that females wish to be molested), and (d) aberrant motivational features such as becoming sexually aroused by photographs of children (Gardner, 2002, 2006; Griffiths, 2002; Reiss & Havercamp, 1997, 1998).

The second grouping of developmentally influenced psychological central processing features would place a person at risk for engaging in SBPs as a result of the *functional absence or low strength* of these features in the person's current skill repertoire. These functional skill deficits increase the risk of SBPs when a person is exposed to conditions of provocation that require the deficit psychological skills as a socially appropriate alternative to the SBPs. Functional skill deficits in such areas as (a) anger management, (b) communication, (c) impulse control, (d) conflict resolution, (e) prosocial alternatives to SBPs, and (f) self-management of prosocial skill alternatives represent illustrations of these central processing features (Baker & Bramston, 1997; Dosen, 2004; Gardner, 2002, 2006; Lindsay, Marshall, Neilson, Quinn, & Smith, 1998).

CONTEXT 3: Maintaining Conditions

Persistently occurring SBPs such as physical and verbal aggression, self-injury, property destruction, and related agitated/disruptive acts often or commonly represent learned behaviors that have become functional in producing various effects of value to the person.

Recurring behavioral challenges become functional in avoiding, delaying, reducing, or terminating experiences of personal distress. The distress may represent conditions of aversive feeling states such pain arising from various physical abnormalities, socially provoked anger, fear, or frustration coupled with physiological overarousal, or fear, anxiety, and irritability created by neurological abnormalities or psychiatric illnesses. The distress also may arise from states of deprivation of such desired experiences as social interaction, personal attention, sensory stimulation, variation in activities, or sexual stimulation. In all instances, the person engages in SBPs as a means of coping with the experienced distressful states of deprivation or overstimulation (Carr, Langdon, & Yarbrough, 1999; Thompson & Symons, 1999). The following provides illustration of this reinforcement process.

> Ms. Jamison, an adult with severe cognitive impairment, a history of physical abuse by her father, and a Posttraumatic Stress Disorder, suddenly became excessively agitated and physically aggressive when a new vocational staff provided physical assistance in completing a difficult work task. The presence of the male with physical features similar to those of her father resulted in noticeable agitation. This personal distress level in combination with the resulting physical touch provided the instigating impetus for the aggressive acts. These aggressive acts resulted in immediate termination of the physical contact and the subsequent removal of the male staff to a different program location. Her aggression as a reaction to this instigating stimulus complex gained in strength as the outburst resulted in reduction in her distressful emotional state.

Neurological Basis of SBPs

Current developments in neuroscience suggest that specific behaviors occur upon activation of particular neuronal circuits within particular brain areas (Kandel, 1998). A neuronal circuit at any particular time represents biological developmental changes, the effects of stress including repeated psychological or physical trauma, and other social experiences of the person. The incoming social experiences may be processed through two different systems of neuronal circuits: subcortical (low road) or cortical (high road) circuit systems (LeDoux, 1996). Some conditions of instigation (e.g., those that are life threatening or highly stressful) as well as experiences during the early years follow the low road and result in an immediate behavioral reaction in the absence of the influence of high cortical mediation. These experiences are stored in the amygdala and usually are rather automatic and not processes consciously. This emotional learning forms neuronal circuits for particular behavior output that occurs beyond cognitive controls (e.g., as in phobias). As the child develops, social experiences gradually are processed with subcortical-cortical influence (high road) by which conscious (cognitive) learning occurs and by which cognitively-mediated neuronal circuits and associated behaviors are formed.

This perspective relating to the different means of neural transmission of antecedent instigating conditions is useful both in understanding the onset mechanism and severity of specific behaviors and in treatment selection. Treatments based on cognitive learning will be less successful than treatment focused on basic emotional needs and motivations for persons who have not demonstrated the developmental features compatible with acquisition of skills involved in cognitive control over behavioral actions. Use of target directed medications in these cases may be useful when used in conjunction with psychological treatment methods (Tyrer, 2001).

Summary: Assessment and Treatment Targets

The initial step in designing suitable treatments and related supports is to identify the conditions that produce and perpetuate personal distress. In the final analysis, successful treatment can be realized only to the extent that the SBPs are viewed and understood from the person's experiential world. Those providing supports for the person will be successful to the extent that they become skillful in detecting what the person is experiencing (i.e., thinking, feeling, perceiving) that renders the serious behavioral acts necessary. Identification of these distress-producing conditions becomes critical in selection of the content and focus of intervention supports provided to reduce the person's distress level. Successful interventions, whether addressing biomedical, psychological, or environmental conditions, will (a) reduce or eliminate the conditions producing the distress and/or (b) teach or strengthen alternatives skills of coping with the distress.

PART B: PRACTICE GUIDELINES

These Practice Guidelines reflect a developmental perspective that is individualized and person-centered and place major emphasis on enhancing the personal competencies of the person presenting with SBPs.

DEVELOPMENTAL PERSPECTIVE. In view of the wide range of developmental impairments present in persons with intellectual disabilities who present SBPs, a developmental perspective guides the diagnostic and treatment selection process. A person's SBPs are best viewed in the context of a person's overall developmental level as well as within specific areas such as cognitive, social, emotional, and personality developmental levels of functioning as these features influence both the manner in which a person interprets and processes relevant instigating conditions as well as the types of SPBs that may be used to cope with these conditions of instigation (Dosen 2005, 2006). Levels of development in specific areas of psychological functioning may differ for a person (e.g., intellectual level may be significantly higher than emotional or social levels) and thus influence the personal meaning for a person of any specific conditions of instigation. As a result, the manner of responding to the instigation may differ.

INDIVIDUALIZED AND PERSON CENTERED PERSPECTIVE. A major focus on respect for the dignity and individuality of each person dictates that assessments and the resulting treatments and related supports be individualized and selected to address the unique set of conditions related to each person's SBPs.

PROGRAM OBJECTIVES: INCREASING PERSONAL COMPETENCIES. The promotion of mental well being, as a major objective, guides service development and delivery. As a result, diagnostic, treatment, management, and related supports are provided as means of promoting mental well being and improving quality of life rather than being undertaken merely to reduce or eliminate a person's SBPs. This objective is accomplished both by providing treatment and related supports designed to increase the person's competencies and by creating increased access to experiences that promote positive social and emotional experiences. Thus, service delivery patterns, locations of service delivery, and interactions of support agency staff are all designed to maximize the positive nature of each for the person, family, and others involved in a person's daily life.

The *Practice Guidelines* are presented in seven sections: An initial section on the Assessment Process (Guideline 1) is followed by sections on Treatment and Related Supports (Guideline 2), Behavioral Crisis Approaches (Guideline 3), Data Systems for Assessment of Treatment Plan Effectiveness (Guideline 4), Types and Contexts of Treatment and Support Plan Services (Guideline 5), Coordination of Services (Guideline 6), and Service Models for Delivery of Services that best serve the needs of persons with SBPs (Guideline 7).

GUIDELINE 1: Comprehensive Biopsychosocial Assessments

Following precise description and definition of an individual's SBPs and a decision that the presenting problems warrant comprehensive treatment and related supports, the next step involves completion of relevant assessments of the various personal and environmental contexts in which these behaviors occur. This assessment process is ongoing and reflects comprehensive attention to the potential multiple biomedical and psychosocial conditions present in the various settings in which the SBPs occur. As such, the assessment is interdisciplinary in nature. Sources of pertinent assessment information include historical and current clinical records, interviews when possible with the person, interviews with relevant informants including family members and care providers, direct behavioral observations within those settings in which the SBPs occur, and a range of more formal and standardized procedures. *These assessments differ in purpose and scope from those undertaken during periods of behavioral crisis. (Refer to Guideline 3).* It is recognized that some referrals for interdisciplinary assessments may be initiated on occurrence of SBPs that represent a danger to self or others or that threaten a current residential placement. In these instances, risk assessments, related crisis management procedures, and crisis planning are undertaken to address the immediate safety needs as the comprehensive assessment process is initiated.

(1a). Purpose and Content of Assessments. A Case Formulation Model that reflects a developmental biopsychosocial (multimodal) approach to understanding SBPs is used to guide the assessment process. This focused information gathering process is designed to identify possible (a) *biomedical* (e.g., physical illness, psychiatric, neuropsychological, medication effects), (b) *psychological, including developmental features (e.g.*, impulse control skills, interpersonal conflict resolution skills, cognitive and language skill levels) and (c) *social and physical environmental* conditions and their interactive effects that contribute to the occurrence, severity levels, variations in occurrence and severity, and persistence of the SBPs. As noted in earlier sections, SBPs are best understood when viewed in the three contexts of *instigating* conditions, *central processing* conditions, and *maintaining* conditions. The manner in which a person will centrally process instigating conditions will reflect the effects of current developmental features of the person. To illustrate, an adult with severely impaired cognitive and related language skills, when angered following peer taunting, will have limited self-managed emotional control and related coping skills available for use in processing the provoking taunts and heightened level of anger. A second adult with a developmental level reflecting mild intellectual disabilities will have the potential for a more complex array of skills with which to process the taunts and to manage a heightened level of anger.

The focus of assessment activities is on (a) identification of the biomedical and psychosocial conditions in each of these three contexts that influence the SBPs of an individual, (b) development of insights into the relative magnitude of effects on the person's SBPs of the various identified influences, and (c) description of the nature of the interactions that occur among the various contributing influences. This assessment process seeks to identify those factors that influence occurrence and persistent recurrence of a person's SBPs as well as those that contribute to the severity levels and variability of these.

To illustrate:

A person's SBP episodes involving physical aggression and self-injurious acts of head banging gradually increased in frequency and

> intensity over a two-month period. On some days, these episodes were noticeably more frequent and intense than on other days. What factors account for the initial base rate, the recent increase in frequency and intensity levels, and the daily variability--Medical influences reflecting physical, psychiatric, or neurological conditions? --Environmental influences? –Psychological influences? How do these separate influences interact?

Insights reflecting possible biopsychosocial conditions are required prior to selecting specific interventions to address these.

The initial step in this process is to obtain descriptive information about the various natural social and physical environmental contexts (home, school, work, day program, etc.) in which behavioral incidents occur. Written or verbal accounts, informal direct observations, checklists, rating scales, and questionnaires, structured interviews, and structured direct observations in the person's natural environments may be used to obtain useful information about potential conditions influencing a person's SBPs in the specific contexts in which these occur.

If conditions identified in the external social, program, and physical settings or in the current physical health status of the person do not provide a suitable account of occurrence, severity levels, and variability of a person's SBPs, more specialized medical (including, psychiatric and neurological) and psychological assessments would be warranted. The most useful information will be obtained relative to possible conditions influencing the person's SBPs when these specialized evaluations are guided by specific inquiries. To illustrate:

> "Within the last month, Ms. G has appeared confused (e.g., has shown periods in which she forgets familiar work routines) and then becomes extremely negativistic (e.g., refuses to follow staff directives and screams at staff) and has become physically aggressive toward staff if again prompted to complete these tasks. These changes in mental state and behaviors appear to coincide with the recent changes in seizure medications. Please give us your opinion about possible

medication effects or other medical conditions that might produce the confusion and related behaviors along with recommendations for medical intervention."

With this referral question, the medical staff will be in a position to provide specific recommendations having treatment relevance to the person's SBPs. (See Guidelines (6b4, 6b5, 6b6) for recommendations relating to the referral process and related supports required.)

(1b). Integration of Assessment Results. Assessments of the conditions that may influence a person's SBPs, and the integration of these data with historical information gained from clinical records and informant reports, would result in a number of hypotheses reflecting multiple modalities (multimodal) of influence (i.e., physical illness conditions, genetic, psychiatric, psychological, and social and physical environmental). As a result of these multiple sources of potential influence, a comprehensive Multimodal Case Formulation format is required to integrate the results of the assessments of the various biomedical and psychosocial modalities of influence into a comprehensive matrix of hypothesized pathological risk conditions. Conditions presumed to produce or contribute to the occurrence, the severity, variability in occurrence and severity, and persistent recurrences of the SBPs are included in the matrix. This comprehensive multimodal approach facilitates an understanding of the separate and possible interactive effects of each set of influences. The Multimodal Contextual Case Formulation Approach described by Gardner (2002) and Gardner and Sovner (1994) provides one example of this approach.

(1c). Composition and Credentials of Assessment Staff. Professionally trained members of community, hospital, and residential service agencies complete assessments relevant to each of the physical illness, psychiatric, psychological, and environmental modalities of influence. These professionals have credentials and clinical practice experiences in:

(1c1). Mental health and developmental disabilities,

(1c2). Assessment and treatment of persons with DD and SBPs,

(1c3). Conducting assessments and devising related interventions programs with consideration given to the developmental status of each person served.

Professionals with these specialty credentials and experiences in medicine, nursing, psychiatry, psychology (including behavior analysis), social work practice, and related specialties (such as speech-language therapists, occupational therapists) are available in a timely manner to provide these assessment and related treatment program development services.

(1d). Setting in Which Assessment and Related Activities Occur. Relevant assessments and the resulting individualized treatment and support services derived from these are provided in environments that are least restrictive and minimally disruptive to the daily living experiences of the person with SBPs. As SBPs, with some infrequent exceptions, are to a major extent influenced in occurrence by antecedents in these daily social and physical environmental settings, diagnostic information relating to these is best obtained within these locations. If behavioral incidents occur in a home setting, evaluation focused on this setting that contains specific social, interpersonal, and physical environmental antecedents, related behavioral consequences, and the interactions of the person with these would occur. If recurring behavioral episodes or even single episodes of major severity occur in the school setting, work setting, or day program settings, as additional examples, diagnostic assessments would focus on these settings in order to understand the **E**nvironment ⇔ **P**erson interactions that in combination determine the occurrences of SBPs. It is these *environments* (home, school, work, day program, and the like) and the *interactions* of the person with specific features of those setting that will become major targets of the treatment and related support services that may ensue.

Although informed clinical practice dictates that the diagnostic process and resulting treatment and related support services be provided in environments that are least intrusive, restrictive, and disruptive to the daily living experiences of the person, it is recognized that various specialized services will be accomplished in various "office" settings. If a physical condition such as recurring headaches is suspected to contribute to a person's distress level that in turn places the person at increased risk for behavioral episodes, medical assessment of these conditions may well be accomplished in a medical office or hospital setting. Even in these instances, the role of any identified medical abnormality in contributing to the person's SBPs can be understood only in the context of the personal distress experienced as a result of the medical condition and the manner in which this experience may interact with other current personal and environmental features. As noted earlier, it is unusual that an occurrence of an SBP would represent the direct and sole result of a medical condition even though in some instances medical conditions may represent a major influence.

In some instances, in view of the severity or chronic occurrence of the SBPs, it may become necessary to remove a person from the community residential setting in which the SBPs occur in order to access respite care or specialty diagnostic and treatment resources. In these instances, it is recognized that the new location becomes a new environment with new expectations, interactions, and related stressors. In many aspects, this placement does not recreate those critical physical environmental and social conditions and routines that influence the person's SBPs in the natural daily settings in which the problems occur. In fact, it is not unusual to observe that the SBPs either do not occur in these new respite or specialty settings or else these occur with greatly reduced frequency and severity. In other instances, as the person is removed from familiar physical and social settings and confronted with new demands and related distress-producing conditions, the SBPs may occur with even greater frequency and severity. The clinical assessment information obtained in these settings thus may be of limited value in identifying, and in detecting the interactive effects of, those salient conditions present in the personal daily social and physical environments in which the behaviors occur and are viewed as a serious problem.

In conclusion, the most relevant diagnostic assessment information will capture those influential conditions that occur in the multiple daily living environments in which the person's SBPs occur. Critical sources of information during the assessment include the person, family, other caregivers, teachers, support staff, or others involved in the daily lives of the person. As noted above, in view of the multiple potential "causes," a *case formulation model* that guides assessments and integrates information obtained is required to reflect the complexity of critical conditions of causation.

GUIDELINE 2. Integrated Treatment and Support Plan.

All biomedical and psychosocial treatments and related supports undertaken to address conditions that influence occurrence and severity of a person's SBPs shall be included in a Comprehensive Individualized Treatment and Support Plan (CITSP). This CITSP is designed specifically to address an individual's needs and personal goals and is based on comprehensive individualized assessment information as described in Guideline 1.

(2a). **Hypothesis-based Interventions**. Each component of the CITSP is hypothesis-driven, that is, designed to address the specific and individually unique complex of instigating, central processing, and maintaining biomedical and psychosocial conditions identified during the assessment process as determinants of the person's SBPs. The CITSP also:

(2a1). Specifies the interrelationships among all components of the Plan, and

(2a2). Includes a process of routinely updating the Plan based on treatment outcomes and new assessment information to insure that the treatments and related supports provided are meeting the current needs of the person served.

(2b). **Content of CITSP**. The CITSP shall include sections devoted to:

(2b1). Proactive approaches that address the antecedent environmental (social, program, physical), psychological, and biomedical instigating conditions under which the SBPs are likely to occur (e.g., excessive noise level, excessive crowding, excessive interpersonal conflict among peers, heightened irritability level associated with untreated allergies, heightened anxiety level),

(2b2). Treatment approaches that address those contingent conditions that serve to strengthen the SBPs,

(2b3). Approaches that support the development and occurrence of developmentally appropriate actions and interactions, with especial attention to those that function as effective alternatives to SBPs.

(2b4). Approaches that insure exposure to habilitatively appropriate physical, social, and program environments that support the individual in accessing opportunities for personal growth and interests, and that insure reasonable freedom from situations that are inconsistent with the individual's current developmental levels and related functioning, skills, or sensitivities. Therapeutic interventions are based on characteristics of the person and avoid exposing the person to interactions that the person finds intolerable or that require adaptation in a manner that is inconsistent with the person's characteristics and needs (e.g., expecting a person with Fragile X syndrome to routinely cope with loud and crowded environments) (Griffiths, Gardner, & Nugent, 1998).

(2b5). Treatment approaches that address relevant biomedical and psychological central processing conditions that contribute to the person's SBPs. Major treatment attention is placed on reducing or eliminating these conditions and on increasing those personal competencies of the person that will replace and thus reduce the functional value of the SBPs, and

(2b6.) Behavioral crisis and deceleration strategies, approaches, and related crisis management guides. This section will highlight conditions and interventions for crisis *prevention* (See Guideline 3).

(2c). **Components of CITSP.** Each component of the CITSP shall:

(2c1). Include objectives and related interventions,

(2c2). Describe the causal relationship between the intervention targets and controlling features of the person's SBPs,

(2c3). Denote the sequence and procedures used to deliver the interventions.

(2c4). Enumerate possible effects and *possible side effects* of the interventions,

(2c5). Describe the procedures used in monitoring the delivery of interventions to insure that these in fact are provided with integrity and consistency in all pertinent settings and

(2c6). Provide guides to insure that interventions are provided for sufficient duration (time period during which intervention effects should be realized) to insure proper evaluation of treatment efficacy,

(2c7). Describe the methods used to evaluate intervention effects and side effects,

(2c9). Specify the staff responsible for reviewing and modifying in a systematic manner the treatment and related support approaches to insure progress and to reflect current needs and related characteristics of the person, and

(2c10). Include specific strategies to insure maintenance and generalization of treatment results beyond the treatment conditions and environments.

(2d). **Empirically-Based Interventions**. The CITSP reflects integration of the most current evidence-based practices with knowledge and expertise acquired through the clinical experiences of team members.

(2d1). These interventions are consistent with the core person-centered values that guide development and implementation of the CITSP,

(2d2). These interventions are nonaversive and minimally intrusive, and

(2d3). Interventions are selected to support (teach and strengthen) personal competencies.

Consistent implementation of this Guideline requires that:

(2d4). Professional staff members who provide the diagnostic and intervention supports, or supervise those who do, shall have routine access to professional literatures and related training opportunities. This is required to insure that staff members are informed about the most current clinical and research findings that offer direction to treatment of the conditions that influence features of a person's SBPs.

GUIDELINE 3: Behavioral Crisis Deceleration Strategies and Crisis Management Supports

As noted in the previous Guideline (2b6), the CITSP includes a specific section in which Deceleration Strategies and Crisis Management (DSCM) supports are described. The goals of the DSCM section of the CITSP include: (a) reducing the emotional or physical distress for the person in the most effective and least intrusive or restrictive manner, (b) insuring protection of others and property, and

(c) terminating the behavioral crisis episode at the earliest possible time consistent with the person's treatment needs (Allen et al., 2001; Davidson et al., 1995; King, Fay, & Croghan, 2000; Zelenski, 2002).

(3a). Content of DSCM. The DSCM section provides description of:

(3a1). Specific individualized adaptations of the person's social or environmental contexts to minimize or eliminate events that may contribute to the SBPs (e.g., disruption of schedules or routines, directives or requests, levels of over- or under-activity),

(3a2). Changes in the person's social interactions or environmental events as a means of promoting specific prosocial behaviors that serve as alternatives to the crisis behaviors,

(3a3). Early behavioral signs previously determined to precede a crisis behavioral episode and, on detection of these,

(3a4). Specific proactive management approaches to follow (e.g., what to do and who does it) in an attempt to reduce or remove influential antecedents,

(3a5). Multiple strategies, including prn or as needed pharmacological strategies, for managing the crisis episode in its various stages (what to do under specific circumstances, who is responsible for implementing and monitoring the effects of various approaches),

(3a6). Specific community service agency responsibilities, including the potential use of police resources,

(3a7). Procedures to follow after resolution of the crisis to debrief and support both the person who was in crisis as well as peers, family, and staff involved,

(3a8). Following resolution of the crisis, treatment strategies to follow at a later time for planned reintroduction of early social-environmental precursors to the crisis as a means of teaching or enhancing coping skills that the person may use on future occasions in response to these or similar conditions.

(3b). Review and Modification of DSCM. The DSCM section of the CITSP shall be modified as needed, following detailed analysis of each crisis occurrence, to insure that the preventive and related treatment approaches and supports are current and do address the conditions identified as contributing to the crisis. Other components of the CITSP will be updated as needed.

(3c). Continuum of Crisis Services in the Natural Environments. The DSCM section of the CITSP includes specific plans for management of a crisis episode in the environment(s) in which the crisis occurs.

When these interventions do not provide for the safety of the person or peers, or for those persons providing initial crisis supports, and when persons supporting the individual in crisis are unable to cope with the behavioral crisis due to its severity or duration, a continuum of additional support service shall be available. The following options should be considered:

(3c1). A mobile cadre of staff, designated in the CITSP, for travel to the settings in which the crisis occurs and to be available in these settings until (a) the crisis attenuates and (b) the person is able to adapt to daily environments, routines, and supports.

(3c2). In those crisis situations that cannot be managed or understood in the person's place of residence or other natural environmental settings in which the crisis occurs (school, vocational, day program), alternative locations shall be available to insure adequate stabilization of a person's acute behavioral, psychological, and psychiatric symptoms. Temporary respites may be offered in a range of settings. These range from placement in:

- A community-based Crisis Respite Residence staffed by support personnel specially trained in treatment and management of individuals with developmental disabilities who present SBPs,
- A specialized short-term stabilization unit in a local hospital,
- A specialized treatment unit in a psychiatric hospital.
- In most communities, admission to these facilities may require an initial assessment in the emergency room of a local general hospital. These emergency room services should be offered education to insure familiarity with practices specifically adapted for persons with intellectual disabilities. See the University of Toronto Guidelines for Management of the Client with Intellectual Disabilities in the Emergency Room) for specific practice recommendations (Bradley, 2002).

(3c3). The least intrusive of the various alternatives shall be used.

(3c4). As soon as safety and acute treatment needs are met, the person shall be returned to his or her place of residence with those supports needed to insure successful reintegration. As much as possible, community support team members should remain involved. This involvement would optimize continuity of care and communication.

GUIDELINE 4: Assessment of CITSP Effectiveness

(4a). Objective Data System. The progress and outcome effectiveness of the separate and combined CITSP components are monitored by use of objective data observation, recording, and evaluation systems. Data based assessment procedures (when reliability and validity concerns have been addressed) would involve standardized scales and inventories as well as individually designed observation and recording procedures.

(4b). Functions of Data Systems. These data systems are used in:

(4b1). Testing hypotheses during case formulation,

(4b2). Supporting the ongoing clinical decision making process, and

(**4b3**). Measuring the impact of individual and combined interventions.

(4c). Ongoing Nature of Assessment. Assessment of progress and outcome effectiveness begins with the initial interventions and is continued as an ongoing process until the treatment objectives have been meet and the treatment and related support program is terminated.

GUIDELINE 5: Comprehensive Individualized Treatment and Related Support Plan Services

(5a). Types of CITSP Services. The following *core* supports shall be provided:

(5a1). Completion of critical assessments, including analysis of possible interpersonal, social, and ecological contributing causes present in the various residential, day program, and other community settings in which a person's SBPs occur,

(5a2). Delivery of critical treatment and related management supports as specified in the CITSP,

(5a3). As needed, crisis interventions in the physical location of the crisis and, when required, in others settings to which the person may be moved to resolve the crisis, and

(5a4). Education, training, and ongoing consultation to existing support resources in the person's daily environments.

(5b). **Contexts of Treatment and Related Support Services.** As SBPs occur in social and ecological contexts as these interact with biomedical and psychological features of the person, core support services will:

(5b1). Be available to the person and significant others requiring supports within the contexts of the natural environments in which the SBPs occur. A *mobile* service team will be required as needed to provide these core support services.

(5b2). Be flexible in nature to meet the treatment and related support needs of the persons supported at specific points in time, and,

(5b3). Use, when feasible, the natural support networks such as family members, staff of residential placements, teachers, and other day program personnel as treatment and related support agents.

(5c). **Targets of CITSP Support Services**. Treatment and related core support services are provided:

(5c1). To the person presenting the SBPs, and

(5c2). To parents, other caregivers or supports staff, teachers, and persons in other natural environments. Ongoing supports provided in the contexts in which the SBPs occur will insure that these persons involved in these environmental and interpersonal contexts are informed about the interactional nature of a person's SBPs.

(5d). **Delivery of CITSP Services.** All treatment and related supports are provided in an individualized and coordinated manner:

(5d1). As detailed in the person's CITSP,

(5d2). With sufficient intensity to insure that interventions reflect the complexity of conditions influencing a person's SBPs,

(5d3.) With consistency across time and in all pertinent settings and conditions, and

(5d4). With sufficient duration to insure that the conditions influencing a person's SBPs are successfully treated or managed.

These guidelines involving intensive and coordinated delivery of services as outlined in the person's CITSP become even more critical, as detailed in Part A, Sections 3, 4, and 5, for those with one or more serious and chronic co-occurring physical illnesses or disorders, genetic syndromes, and psychiatric disorders.

GUIDELINE 6: Coordination of Treatment and Related Support Services

(6a). Treatment Plan Coordinator. A Treatment Plan Coordinator skilled and experienced in implementing a Multimodal Case Formulation approach shall be available to insure delivery of coordinated treatment and related supports as specified in the CITSP.

(6b). Functions of Treatment Plan Coordinator. The Treatment Plan Coordinator or, when needed, a designated alternate who is thoroughly familiar with the specifics of the person and the CITSP assumes responsibility to:

(6b1). Insure the full integration of the separate components of the CITSP,

(6b2). Facilitate timely and coordinated delivery of treatment and support services as detailed in a person's CITSP,

(6b3). As the CITSP is dynamic and subject to change, insure that the CITSP is updated as new information is obtained and insure that all relevant persons are informed of these updates,

(6b4). When referral is made for specific assessment, treatment, and related support services, facilitate the referral process by preparing the person (and family members when relevant) for participation in the assessment and treatment process,

(6b5). As needed, accompany the person and family or caregiver to the assessment, treatment, and related support service referral appointments.

This coordinator function is especially significant when the professionals providing specific assessment, treatment, or related support services are not familiar with the person or else have minimal familiarity with persons with developmental disabilities. The objective of this coordinator function is to enhance communication to:

- Insure that the professional staff providing the specific service(s) is fully informed about the referral question(s),
- Support the person in communicating his or her concerns and the specific information requested by the professional staff, and
- Insure that comprehensive pertinent information about the person and the SBPs is current and is appropriately communicated to the professional staff providing the requested professional services. This Treatment Coordinator function would insure that current relevant information is available and that the professional staff members providing services are completely informed about the referral questions. Information would include a succinct summary of pertinent history and a detailed presentation of current information relevant to the assessment and/or treatment issues.

(6b6). Following completion of the referral, report the results to the treatment team to insure that all treatment and related support staff and family are provided complete and current information.

(6b7). Coordinate rapid response to behavioral crisis.

(6c) **Caseload of Treatment Plan Coordinator.** The size of the caseload of the Treatment Plan Coordinator will be determined by the individual support requirements of the persons served by a specific Coordinator. Caseload size should permit sufficient contact with the support recipients (i.e., the person presenting the SBPs and with those who provide routine supports for this individual in his or her natural environments) of sufficient frequency and duration to:

(6c1). Insure development of a trusting relationship or partnership,

(6c2). Permit sufficient ongoing contacts to insure that the person's treatment and related support needs are being met in a timely manner,

(6c3). Insure coordination of intensive services for each person served,

(6c4). Insure integration of services in complex cases,

(6c5). Insure adequate communication between the person and family members with the treatment team and consulting professionals and programs, and

(6c6). Insure rapid response to behavioral crises.

(6d). Duration of Services of Treatment Plan Coordinator. Services of the Treatment Plan Coordinator for persons with SBPs, although differing in type and intensity depending on the treatment and related support needs of a person and family at any given time, should be:

(6d1). Available in a timely manner whenever the need arises to provide individualized supports. As critical problems may occur after typical office hours, including nights and weekends, Treatment Plan Coordinator work schedules are structured to insure that needs are meet in a timely manner.

(6d2). Ongoing over the duration of time in which SPBs are present. In view of the chronic and recurring nature of some SBPs, and of the conditions that influence their occurrence such as chronic psychiatric and other recurring medical conditions, the need of some individuals for Treatment Plan Coordinator services may extend over a significant segment of the person's life span.

GUIDELINE 7: Approaches to Delivery of Core and Related Services

(7a). **Service Agency or Consortium of Service Agencies.** A service agency or a consortium of service agencies is designated to deliver a specific service or a set of core and related services.

(7b). **Seamless Service Delivery.** The service agency or consortium of service agencies involved provides integrated, coordinated, and seamless service delivery as needed over the life span of persons served.

(7c). **Specific Responsibility for Coordination of Services.** If a consortium of core and related support services agencies is utilized, a designated program or agency within the consortium is given specific responsibility to insure that the separate services are in fact integrated, coordinated, and seamless in meeting the needs of the persons served.

(7d). Services and Roles. The core agency or consortium of service agencies, in addition to commitment to the guiding principles detailed in the Overview section, includes the following services and roles:

(7d1). Multimodal assessments, (See Guideline 1),

(7d2). Specialized treatment and related support resources (See Guidelines 2, 3, 4, and 5),

(7d3). Specialized intensive support and program coordination services (See Guideline 6),

(7d4). Specialty consultations to generic community and regional mental health, health, education, and social and family support agencies who may provide agency related services to persons with developmental disabilities who present with SBPs,

(7d5). Training opportunities for professionals in generic mental health, health, education, and social and family support agencies in identification, treatment, and management of SBPs and related topics relevant to persons with developmental disabilities,

(7d6). Training opportunities for family and other support personnel in prevention, early identification, management of SBPs, and related topics,

(7d7). Information dissemination relating to SBPs.

(7d8). Quality assurance and program effectiveness assessment process to insure ongoing QA monitoring and timely program modification as needed.

Summary

Description has been provided of features of SBPs that require specialized and individualized supports services. Additionally, sets of Practice Guidelines that address the types of services, personnel, and agency structures required are described. These Guidelines to practice are grounded in core values that guide support service development and delivery. The major objective of person-centered treatment and related support services is that of promoting mental wellness and related personal coping as alternatives to SBPs. This emphasis shifts the major focus from one of identification and management of sources of pathology to a focus of increasing a person's quality of life through promotion of personal competencies and related mental wellness.

References

Allen, M. H., Currier, G. W., Hughes, D. H., Reyes-Harde, M, Docherty, J. P., & Ross, G. W. (2001). Treatment of behavioral emergencies. Expert Consenses Guideline Series. Postgraduate Medicine Special Report. May 2001. White Plains, NY: Expert Knowledge Systems.

Anderson, J. T., & Ernst, M. (1994). Self-injury in Lesch Nyhan disease. Journal of Autism and Developmental Disorders 24, 67-82.

Baker, W., & Bramston, P. (1997). Attributional and emotional determinants of aggression in people with mild intellectual disabilities. Journal of Intellectual and Developmental Disabilities, 22, 169-186.

Barnhill, J. (1999). The relationships between epilepsy and violent behavior in persons with mental retardation. The NADD Bulletin, 2, 43-46.

Barnhill, J. (2001). Behavioral phenotypes: A glimpse into the neuropsychiatry of genes (Part II): Analysis of behavioral phenotypes-social anxiety in Fragile X syndrome and autism. The NADD Bulletin, 4, 63-69.

Bouras, N., & Drummond, C. (1992). Behavior and psychiatric disorders of people with mental handicaps living in the community. Journal of Intellectual Disability Research, 36, 349-357.

Bradley, E. (2002). Guidelines for managing the client with intellectual disability in the emergency room. Toronto: Centre for Addiction and Mental Health, University of Toronto.

Bradley, S. J. (2000). Affect regulation and the development of psychopathology. New York: The Guilford Press.

Brylewski, J., & Wiggs, L. (1999). Sleep problems and daytime challenging behaviour in a community-based sample of adults with intellectual disability. Journal of Intellectual Disability Research, 43, 504-512.

Carr, E. G., Langdon, N. A., & Yarbrough, S. C. (1999). Linking functional assessment to effective intervention. In A. C. Repp & R. H. Horner, (Eds.), Functional analysis of problem behavior (pp. 7-31). Belmont, CA: Wadsworth.

Cole, C. L., & Gardner, W. I. (1990). Effects of staff- and self-assessment procedures on disruptive behaior in a vocational setting: A case study. Vocational Evaluation and Work Assessment Bulletin, 23, 41-46.

Comings, D. E., & Comings, B. G. (1985). Tourette syndrome: Clinical and psychological aspects of 250 cases. American Journal of Human Genetics, 37, 435-450.

Creaby, M., Warner, M., Jamil, N., & Jawad, S. (1993). Ictal aggression in severely mentally handicapped people. Irish Journal of Psychological Medicine, 10, 12-15.

Davidson, P. W., Caine, N. N., Sloane-Reeves, J. E., Gresow, V. E., Quigano, L. E., Vanlteyningen, J., & Shoham, I. (1995). Crisis intervention for community-based individuals with developmental disabilities and behavioral and psychiatric disorders. Mental Retardation, 33, 21-33.

Dosen, A. (2004). The developmental psychiatric approach to aggressive behaviors among persons with mental retardation. Mental Health Aspects of Developmental Disabilities, 57-68.

Dosen, A. (2005a). Applying the developmental perspective in the psychiatric assessment and diagnosis of persons with intellectual disabilities. Part I: Assessment. Journal of Intellectual Disabilities Research, 49(1), 1-8.

Dosen, A. (2005b). Applying the developmental perspective in the psychiatric assessment and diagnosis of persons with intellectual disability. Part II: Diagnosis. Journal of Intellectual Disabilities Research, 49(1), 9-15.

Dykens, E. M. (1996). DNA meets DSM: The growing importance of genetic syndromes in dual diagnosis. Mental Retardation, 34, 125-127.

Dykens, E. M., Hodapp, R. M., & Finucane, B. M. (2000). Genetics and mental retardation syndromes. Baltimore: Paul H. Brookes Publishing.

Einfeld, S. I., Tonge, B. J., & Florio, T. (1997). Behavioral and emotional disturbance in individuals with Williams syndrome. American Journal of Mental Retardation, 102, 45-53.

Emerson, E. (2001). Challenging behaviour. Analysis and intervention in people with learning difficulties. Cambridge University Press, Cambridge.

Forehand, R., & Wierson, M, (1993). The role of developmental factors in planning behavioral interventions for children: Disruptive behavior as an example. Behavior Therapy, 24, 117-141.

Friedman, D. L., Kastner, T., Plummer, A. T., Ruiz, M. Q., & Henning, D. (1992). Adverse behavioral effects in individuals with mental retardation and mood disorders treated with carbamazepine. American Journal of Mental Retardation, 96, 541-546..

Gardner, W. I. (2002). Aggression and other disruptive behavioral challenges: Biomedical and psychosocial assessment and treatment. Kingston, NY: NADD Press.

Gardner, W. I., & Hunter, R. H. (2003). Psychosocial diagnosis and treatment services in inpatient psychiatric facilities for persons with mental retardation: Practice Guides. Mental Health Aspects of Developmental Disabilities, 6, 68-80.

Gardner, W. I., & Sovner, R. (1994). Self-injurious behaviors: Diagnosis and treatment. Willow Street, PA: Vida Press.

Gardner, W. I., & Whalen, J. P. (1996). A multimodal behavior analytic model for evaluating the effects of medical problems on nonspecific behavioral symptoms in persons with developmental disabilities. Behavioral Interventions, 11, 147-161.

Gedye, A. (1997). Behavioral diagnostic guide for developmental disabilities. Vancouver: Diagnostic Books.

Greenspan, S. J. (1997). Developmentally based psychotherapy. Madison: International University Press.

Griffiths, D. M. (2002). Sexual aggression. In W. I. Gardner, Aggression and other disruptive behavioral challenges: Biomedical and psychosocial assessment and treatment (pp. 325-397). Kingston, NY: NADD Press.

Griffiths, D. M., & Gardner, W. I. (2002a). Programs and intervention approaches for the treatment of persons with dual diagnosis: A summary. In J. W. Jacobson, S. Holburn, & J. A. Mulick (Eds.), Contemporary dual diagnosis: MH/MR. Service models Vol II: Partial and supportive services (pp. 141-149). Kingston, NY: The NADD Press.

Griffiths, D. M., & Gardner, W. I. (2002b). Residential and day programs for persons with dual diagnosis: A summary. In J. W. Jacobson, S. Holburn, & J. A. Mulick (Eds.), Contemporary dual diagnosis: MH/MR. Service models Vol I: Residential and day services (pp. 123-139). Kingston, NY: The NADD Press.

Griffiths, D. M., Gardner, W. I., & Nugent, J.A. (1998). Behavioral supports: Individual centered interventions. Kingston, NY: NADD Press.

Griffiths, D., & King, R. (2004). Demystifying syndromes: Clinical and educational implications of common syndromes associated with persons with intellectual disabilities. Kingston, NY: NADD Press.

Griffiths, D., & Watson, S. L. (2004). Demystifying syndromes associated with developmental disabilities, In D. Griffiths & R. King, Demystifying syndromes: Clinical and educational implications of common syndromes associated with persons with intellectual disabilities (pp. 1-30).Kingston, NY: NADD Press.

Griffiths, D. M., Stavrakaki, & Summers, J. (Eds.). (2002). Dual diagnosis: An introduction to the mental health needs of persons with developmental disabilities. Sudsbury, Ontario: Habilitative Mental Health Resource Network.

Harris, J. C. (1998). Developmental neuropsychiatry, Vol II. Oxford: Orford University Press.

Jacobson, J. W., Holburn, S., & Mulick, J. A. (Eds.). (2002). Contemporary dual diagnosis: MH/MR service models Vol II: Partial and supportive services. Kingston, NY: The NADD Press.

Jacobson, J. W., Mulick, J. A., & Holburn, S. (Eds.). (2002). Contemporary dual diagnosis: MH/MR service models Vol I: Residential and day services. Kingston, NY: The NADD Press.

Kalachnik, J. E., Hanzel, T. E., Harder, S. R., Bauernfeind, J. D., & Engstromn, E. A. (1995). Antiepileptic drug behavioral side effects in individuals with mental retardation and the use of behavioral measurement techiques. Mental Retardation, 33, 374-382.

Kandel, E. R. (1998). A new intellectual framework of psychiatry. American Journal of Psychiatry, 155(4), 457-469.

King, R. (1999). Comorbidity in Tourette's syndrome: Pharmacological treatment in adults with a severe to profound handicap. The NADD Bulletin, 2, 3-7.

King, R., Fay, G., & Croghan, P. (2000). Pro Re Nata: Optimal use of psychotropic PRN medication. Mental Health Aspects of Developmental Disabilities, 3, 8-16.

Lakin, K. C., & Larson, S. A. (2002). The social and policy context of community-centered behavioral supports and crisis response. In R. H. Hanson, N. A. Wieseler, & K. C. Lakin (Eds.), Crisis: Prevention and response in the community (pp. 3-32). Washington, DC: American Association on Mental Retardation.

LeDoux, J. (1996). The emotional brain. New York: Simon & Schuster.

Lindsay, W. H., Marshall, I., Neilson, C. Quinn, K., & Smith, A. H. W. (1998). The treatment of a person with a learning disability convicted of exhibitionism. Research in Developmental Disabilities, 19, 295-316..

McComas, J., Hoch, H., Paone, D., & El-Roy, D. (2000). Escape behavior during academic tasks: A preliminary analysis of idiosyncratic establishing operations. Journal of Applied Behavior Analysis, 33, 479-493.

Moss, S. C., Emerson, E., Kierman, C., Turner, S., Hatton, C., & Alborz, A. (2000). Psychiatric symptoms in adults with learning diability and challenging behaviour. British Journal of Psychiatry, 177, 452-456.

O'Brien, G. (2003). The classification of problem behaviour in Diagnostic Criteria for Psychiatric Disorders for Use with Adults with Learning Disabilities/Mental Retardation (DC-LD). Journal of Intellectual Disability Research, 47, 32-37.

O'Reilly, M. F. (1995). Functional analysis and treatment of escape-maintained aggression correlated with sleep deprivation. Journal of Applied Behavioral Analysis, 28, 225-226.

Pary, R. J. (2005). The referral dilemma of challenging behaviors, psychiatric disorders, and treatment. Are there shortcuts in 2005? Mental Health Aspect of Developmental Disabilities, 8, 126-128.

Peine, H. A., Darvish, R., Adams, K., Blakelock, H. M., Jenson, W., & Osborne, J. G. (1995). Medical problems, maladaptive behaviors, and the developmentally disabled. Behavioral Interventions, 10, 149-159.

Reiss, S. (1992). Assessment of a man with a dual diagnosis. Mental Retardation, 30, 1-6.

Reiss, R., & Aman, M. G. (Eds.). (1998). Psychotropic medication and developmental disabilities: The international consensus handbook. Ohio State University Nisonger Center. Columbus, Ohio.

Reiss, S., & Havercamp, S. M. (1997). Sensitivity theory and mental retardation: Why functional analysis is not enough. American Journal of Mental Retardation, 101, 553-566.

Reiss, S., & Havercamp, S. M. (1998). Toward a comprehensive assessment of fundamental motivation: Factor structure of the Reiss Profiles. Psychological Assessment, 10, 97-106.

Richardson, S. A., Koller, H., & Katz, M. (1985). Continuities and change in behavior disturbance: A follow-up study of mildly mentally retarded young people. American Journal of Orthopsychiatry, 55, 220-229.

Reed, G. M., McLaughlin, J., & Newman, R. (2002). The development and evaluation of guidelines for professional practice. American Psychologist, 57, 1041-1047.

Robertson, M., Trimble, M., & Lees, A. (1989). Self-injurious behavior and the Gilles de la Tourette syndrome: A clinical study and review of the literature. Psychological Medicine, 19, 611-625.

Rush, J., & Frances, A. (Eds.) (2002). Expert Consensus Guidelines Series: Treatment of psychiatric and behavioral problems in mental retardation. American Journal of Mental Retardation, 105, 1-228.

Ryan, R. (1994). Posttraumatic stress disorders in persons with developmental disabilities. Community Mental Health Journal, 30, 45-54.

Ryan, R. (2000). Posttraumatic stress disorder in persons with developmental disabilities. In A. Poindexter (Ed.), Assessment and treatment of anxiety disorders in persons with mental retardation: revised and updated for 2000 (pp. 37-45). Kingston, NY: NADD Press.

Sovner, R., Foxx, C. J., Lowry, M. J., & Lowry, M. A. (1993). Fluoretine treatment of depression and associated self-injury in two adults with mental retardation. Journal of Intellectual Disabilities Research, 37,301-311.

Thompson, T., & Symons, F. J. (1999). Neobehavioral mechanisms of drug action. In N. A. Wieseler & R. H. Hanson (Eds.), Challenging behavior of persons with mental health disorders and severe developmental disabilities (pp 125-150). Washington, DC: American Association on Mental Retardation.

Tsiouris, J. A. (2001). Diagnosis of depression in people with severe/profound mental disabilities. Journal of Intellectual Disabilities Research, 45, 115-120.

Tu, J., Shafey, H., & VanDewetering, C. (1994). Iron deficiency in two adolescents with conduct dysthymic and movement disorders. Canadian Journal of Psychiatry, 39, 371-375.

Tucker, G. J., Price, T. R., Johnson, V. B., & McAllister, T. (1986). Phenomenology of temporal lobe dyusfunction. A link to atypical psychosis - a series of cases. Journal of Nervous and Mental Disease, 174, 348-356.

Tuinier, S., & Verhoeven, W. M. A. (1993). Psychiatry and mental retardation: Towards a behavioural pharmacological concept. Journal of Intellectual Disability Research 37, 16-25.

Tyrer, S. (2001). Psychopharmacological approaches. In A. Dosen & K. Day (eds.), Treating mental illness and behavior disorders in children and adults with mental retardation (pp. 45-68). Washington, DC: American Psychiatry Press.

Vitiello, B., Speat, S., & Behar, D. (1989). Obsessive-compulsive disorder in mentally retarded patients. Journal of Nervous and Mental Disease, 177, 232-236.

Vitiello, B., & Stoff, D. M. (1997). Subtypes of aggression and their relevance to child psychiatry. Journal of American Academy of Child and Adolescent Psychiatry, 36,307-315.

Zelenski, S. (2002). Evaluation for and use of psychopharmacologic treatment in crisis intervention for people with mental retardation and mental illness. In R. H. Hanson, N. A. Wieseler, & K. C. Lakin (Eds.), Crisis: Prevention and response in the community (pp. 243-256). Washington, DC: American Association on Mental Retardation.